GUA SHA FOR BEGINNERS

Step-By-Step Guide To Facial And Body Scraping Techniques For Pain Relief, Skin Rejuvenation, And Enhanced Wellbeing

DR SAWYER DIEGO

DISCLAMER

Nothing in this book should be interpreted as medical advice; it is meant exclusively for educational reasons. Regarding their specific health issues and treatment options, readers are urged to speak with licensed healthcare professionals. The publisher and author disclaim all liability for any errors or omissions in the material provided, as well as for any negative effects that may arise from using or abusing the information. Although every attempt has been taken to guarantee that the material in this book is correct as of the date of publishing, new research may have superseded some of the content because medical knowledge is always changing. It is recommended that readers confirm the most recent medical recommendations and guidelines. The reader of this book undertakes to release the author and publisher from any claims or liabilities resulting from the use of this information, and understands and accepts the inherent risks connected with healthcare decisions.

TABLE OF CONTENTS

ABOUT THE BOOK

The book "Gua Sha for Beginners" offers a thorough introduction to the history, advantages, methods, and real-world applications of this age-old healing art, making it an indispensable resource for anybody interested in learning more. Gua Sha, which has its roots in traditional Chinese medicine (TCM), uses a variety of tools and mild scraping techniques to enhance well-being holistically. Knowing its history and the fundamentals of TCM not only broadens one's understanding but also helps one appreciate its therapeutic possibilities.

The examination of Gua Sha's many advantages—from pain alleviation and better circulation to enhanced skin health and stress reduction—is at the heart of the book. By exploring these advantages, readers can learn how to incorporate Gua Sha into their wellness regimens to support mental and physical well-being via improved lymphatic drainage and natural cleansing processes.

A recurrent topic is the significance of correct technique, which highlights safety concerns, dispels myths, and helps readers set reasonable expectations. By providing comprehensive guidance on selecting appropriate instruments, readying the skin, and grasping both fundamental and sophisticated methods, the book enables novices to incorporate Gua Sha into their everyday routines with ease.

Furthermore, answering often-asked questions and resolving common issues guarantees a complete comprehension of Gua Sha's safety and effectiveness, allaying worries about bruising or negative side effects. For individuals looking to advance their practice, advanced procedures and specialized equipment are explored. These include creative applications like combining acupuncture with Gua Sha or boosting facial rejuvenation treatments with serums and essential oils.

Looking ahead, the book highlights new tools and methodologies, technological integrations, and worldwide perspectives on the influence of Gua Sha, anticipating future trends and advances in the field. The book invites readers to interact with this age-old activity thoughtfully and progressively by promoting an awareness of sustainable production processes for Gua Sha.

"Gua Sha for Beginners" is essentially more than just a manual; it's a doorway to unlocking the life-changing possibilities of gua sha. It provides insightful and useful advice that opens doors to long-term health and holistic self-care.

CHAPTER ONE
GUA SHA OVERVIEW
GUA SHA DEFINITION

Gua Sha is an age-old healing method derived from traditional Chinese medicine that involves using a massage tool to scrape the skin to increase circulation. The word "Gua Sha" means "scraping sand," and it describes the redness (petechiae) that occurs on the skin following treatment and resembles sand. This technique seeks to increase blood flow, soothe tense muscles, and discharge qi, or stagnant energy. Usually done using instruments made of jade, rose quartz, or buffalo horn, gua sha is a mild yet powerful treatment that can be used on the back, neck, arms, and legs.

The method uses long or short strokes to scrape the skin, depending on the area being treated and the desired outcome, while gently applying pressure. It's frequently used to promote lymphatic drainage, lessen inflammation, and ease muscle discomfort and tightness. Gua Sha may temporarily create redness or bruises, but these are good indicators of improved circulation and toxin elimination. The method has its roots in the Chinese medical theory that maintains total health and well-being by balancing the body's energy.

Gua Sha's renown goes beyond that of traditional Chinese medicine, becoming ingrained in contemporary wellness regimens across the globe. It is accessible to novices looking for natural ways to improve their health and energy because of its simplicity and efficiency. People can effectively support physical and emotional wellness by incorporating Gua Sha into their self-care routines by knowing its fundamental concepts and procedures.

ADVANTAGES OF GUA SHA

Gua Sha has advantages that go beyond simple relaxation; it can enhance mental and physical health. Its capacity to increase circulation can assist lessen muscular stiffness and increase flexibility, which is one of its main benefits. Gua Sha helps the body's natural healing processes by speeding up the removal of metabolic waste products and promoting blood flow, which helps supply oxygen and nutrients to tissues.

Gua Sha is also well renowned for its ability to relieve chronic pain, especially in the lower back, shoulders, and neck. The mild scraping motion of the method relieves discomfort and encourages relaxation by releasing tension that has been stored in the muscles and fascia.

Additionally, by boosting collagen formation and diminishing the appearance of fine lines and wrinkles, regular Gua Sha treatments may aid in the improvement of skin health.

Beyond its physical advantages, Gua Sha promotes mental and emotional health by fostering a profound sense of relaxation. The repetitive scraping actions have the potential to improve mood, lower stress levels, and promote mental calmness.

Gua Sha is a flexible technique appropriate for people looking for natural ways to improve their quality of life because of its holistic approach to wellness.

HOW GUA SHA CAN ENHANCE YOUR HEALTH

Gua Sha treats the physical as well as the energetic components of health, providing a comprehensive approach to enhancing general well-being. Gua Sha encourages circulation by gently scraping the body, which is necessary for carrying nutrients and oxygen throughout the body and eliminating waste products and toxins from metabolism. In addition to aiding the body's natural healing processes, this improved circulation also helps release tightness and tension in the muscles.

Gua Sha can also have a significant impact on the lymphatic system, which is essential for the immune system and detoxification processes. Gua Sha helps eliminate extra fluid and encourages a healthy flow of lymphatic fluid throughout the body by inducing lymphatic drainage. This can boost general vigor, strengthen the immune system, and lessen edema.

Apart from its physiological advantages, traditional Chinese medicine regards Gua Sha for its capacity to harmonize the body's energy channels. Gua Sha helps to enhance mental clarity and emotional well-being by facilitating the smooth flow of energy and clearing stagnant qi.

People who practice regularly report feeling more resilient, calm and grounded when handling daily stressors.

THE SIGNIFICANCE OF USING THE RIGHT METHOD

The correct use of technique, which emphasizes light yet deliberate scraping strokes across the skin, is crucial to the efficacy of Gua Sha. It's important to use the proper kind of tool, which is usually made of materials like rose quartz or jade and glides over the skin easily without inflicting pain or damage. To get the best outcomes, the tool's pressure and angle should be changed based on the body part being treated and its sensitivity.

Understanding the direction of strokes, which varies based on the desired result, is another aspect of proper technique. For instance, horizontal or circular motions may be more appropriate for relieving muscle tension in the neck and shoulders than vertical strokes, which are frequently employed to encourage lymphatic drainage on the back. The intention is to ensure that the patient has a favorable experience by producing a gentle scraping sensation that feels therapeutic rather than painful.

In addition, it's crucial to follow good hygiene when doing Gua Sha to avoid infections or skin irritation. To ensure smooth tool gliding, the skin should be sufficiently hydrated or lubricated with oil. Tools should also be cleaned completely before and after each usage. To fully benefit from Gua Sha, people can safely incorporate it into their self-care routines by emphasizing good technique and hygiene.

CHAPTER TWO
COMPREHENDING GUA SHA
THE ORIGINS AND HISTORY OF GUA SHA

Traditional Chinese medicine (TCM) gave rise to the age-old healing method known as gua sha, which has a long history that dates back thousands of years. Its origins can be found in rural China and Southeast Asia, where practitioners utilized smooth-edged implements to scrape the skin's surface to treat a variety of diseases. The word "Gua Sha" itself means "scraping sand" in Chinese, highlighting the practice's historical application of scraping to expel heat and toxins thought to be trapped in the body.

With time, Gua Sha transcended its local roots and gained international recognition as a treatment for improving general health, decreasing inflammation, and increasing circulation. Its historical relevance stems from its incorporation into Traditional Chinese Medicine (TCM), where it was and is used as a means of qi (vital energy) balance and health maintenance.

Because of its versatility, the technique has been widely adopted by many cultures, each of which has given it distinctive customs while maintaining its core values of promoting circulation and assisting the body's natural healing processes.

Gua Sha is still popular today because of its holistic approach to health, cultural history, and therapeutic effects. Its rise in current wellness practices highlights its ongoing relevance and usefulness in addressing contemporary health issues by fusing traditional knowledge with new insights into human physiology.

TRADITIONAL CHINESE MEDICINE'S (TCM) FUNDAMENTALS

The fundamental ideas of traditional Chinese medicine (TCM), which sees health as a balance of yin and yang energy within the body, are essential to Gua Sha's practice. TCM theory states that disease results from disturbances in the blood and qi flow along meridians or energy channels.

Gua Sha is used to clear stagnation, encourage qi flow, and expel built-up heat and toxins from the body to bring this flow back.

The method is lightly scraping the skin's surface with an instrument, usually made of pottery, buffalo horn, or jade, utilizing precise strokes. The "sha" or redness on the skin is the result of these strokes that are made along the meridians or in specific uncomfortable spots. This sha is thought to disappear when circulation improves, revitalizing the skin and encouraging internal healing. It is seen as a visible sign of blood stagnation.

Gua Sha practitioners follow TCM concepts to treat underlying imbalances in the body's energy flow in addition to physical problems. With a focus on prevention and repair, this holistic approach sees the body as a networked system in which outward manifestations of health, such as skin tone and appearance, are reflections of underlying health issues.

People can incorporate Gua Sha into their wellness practices to promote general health and energy by comprehending these concepts.

VARIOUS GUA SHA TOOL TYPES

Gua Sha implements are made of different materials and have different forms, each with its own advantages and healing powers. In the past, natural materials with smooth edges and durability, like jade, bone, or horn, were used to manufacture tools. These substances not only made scraping more efficient, but they also added warmth or cooling qualities that enhanced Gua Sha's healing effects.

Gua Sha instruments are still in use today, but they come in plastic, stainless steel, and rose quartz varieties to suit a variety of tastes and therapeutic purposes. Smooth-edged instruments are the best choice since they provide controlled pressure and efficient circulation stimulation while ensuring gentle scraping without abrasions. The size and form of each sort of tool can differ, ranging from larger instruments appropriate for larger body parts to small gadgets with several edges for adaptability.

When choosing a Gua Sha tool, factors such as material qualities, intended application, and personal comfort should be taken into account. Wider tools work well for covering wider areas, such as the back or limbs, whereas instruments with curved or pointed edges may be chosen for targeting certain acupoints or muscle groups. By being aware of these differences, people can select a tool that best meets their requirements, increasing the effectiveness and satisfaction of their Gua Sha practice.

SAFETY OBSERVATIONS AND SAFETY MEASURES

Even while gua sha is generally safe when done properly, practitioners should follow important safety guidelines to optimize its advantages and reduce any possible concerns. The most important thing to remember when scraping is to make sure the tool's edges are smooth and devoid of sharp edges or nicks to avoid causing injuries to the skin. To maintain hygiene, it's best to use equipment made of non-porous materials that are simple to clean and disinfect in between uses.

The pressure used during scraping is another crucial factor to take into account. Using too much force might hurt or bruise, especially on delicate or thin skin areas. It is recommended that practitioners begin with mild pressure and progressively increase it as necessary, observing the skin's and body's response. It is imperative to steer clear of damaged or irritated skin areas to avoid aggravating pre-existing conditions or allowing infections to enter open wounds.

In addition, before doing Gua Sha, practitioners with certain medical concerns, such as blood disorders, skin sensitivities, or recent surgeries, should speak with healthcare providers. Women who are expecting should use caution, concentrating on soft methods and avoiding areas around their abdomens. People can comfortably incorporate Gua Sha into their health routines and properly and efficiently utilize its therapeutic effects by emphasizing safety and awareness throughout practice.

FREQUENTLY HELD MYTHS REGARDING GUA SHA

There are a few common misconceptions about gua sha, even if its popularity is rising, which can discourage people from learning more about its advantages. The transitory redness or sha that emerges on the skin during scraping is a normal physiological response and usually goes away in a few days. It is a frequent misconception that gua sha causes bruises or skin injury. This sha is a sign of better circulation and toxin release rather than bruise.

There is also a misperception that Gua Sha is uncomfortable or painful. When done correctly, with the right pressure and skill, gua sha should be calming and stimulating, encouraging relaxation and the release of tense muscles.

Practitioners can customize the experience to their comfort level by varying the tool's pressure and angle, which guarantees a good and joyful session.

Furthermore, some people might think that gua sha is just a cosmetic procedure. Although it can improve the appearance of the skin by encouraging lymphatic drainage and circulation, its main advantages are in bolstering general health and wellbeing by restoring blood flow and qi. People can confidently embrace the comprehensive advantages of Gua Sha by clearing up these myths and realizing that it's a therapeutic technique with roots in ancient healing traditions.

CHAPTER THREE
ADVANTAGES OF GUA SHA
RELAXATION OF THE MUSCLES AND PAIN RELIEF

The traditional Chinese medicinal method known as gua sha is incredibly beneficial for reducing pain and relaxing muscles. A smooth-edged instrument, like a jade or rose quartz gua sha tool, can be used to gently scrape the skin to encourage microcirculation in the soft tissue. This motion is especially useful for relieving muscle pain and stiffness following physical exercise or extended periods of tension since it helps to release tension and tightness in the muscles. In addition to promoting the release of endorphins, the body's natural painkillers, gua sha's mild pressure also helps to reduce discomfort and enhance well-being.

Because gua sha reduces inflammation and increases blood flow to the affected areas, regular treatments can considerably improve flexibility and mobility.

By focusing on trigger points and knots in the muscles, the technique encourages relaxation and restores the natural harmony of muscular tone. The body feels relief from chronic pain disorders such as lower back pain, neck pain, and tension headaches as the muscles relax.

Beginners should always use light pressure at first and raise it gradually as comfort permits. This will guarantee a soothing, yet gentle, experience that improves relaxation and supports the health of your muscles in general.

Before doing gua sha, it is advised to lubricate the skin with a natural oil or lubricant to minimize friction and improve the tool's smooth glide. Pay particular attention to the shoulders, neck, and lower back, as these are areas that are commonly tense and uncomfortable. Make slow, methodical movements in a single direction, adhering to the muscles' natural curves. Rest and drink plenty of water after a workout to aid in your body's healing. Beginners can successfully utilize gua sha's benefits for pain treatment and muscular relaxation, promoting a holistic approach to well-being, with regular practice.

IMPROVED LYMPHATIC DRAINAGE AND CIRCULATION

Gua sha treatment has a great deal to offer in terms of lymphatic drainage and circulation improvement, both of which are essential for preserving general health and energy. The method, which involves lightly scraping the skin's surface, increases blood flow to the treated area, facilitating the supply of nutrients and oxygen to the tissues. By removing toxins and metabolic waste, this improved circulation lowers inflammation and aids in the body's natural healing processes. Enhancing blood circulation also helps to maintain a more youthful-looking complexion by improving skin tone and texture.

Apart from augmenting blood circulation, gua sha encourages lymphatic drainage, which facilitates the elimination of lymphatic fluid accumulation and diminishes facial and body edema.

Started lymphatic fluid is moved toward lymph nodes by the gentle scraping movement, where it can be filtered and expelled from the body. In addition to cleansing the skin, this procedure strengthens the immune system, promoting general health and lowering the chance of infection. Gua sha can help beginners achieve a clearer, more vibrant complexion and increase the effectiveness of their body's detoxification processes when added to their skincare regimen.

To achieve the best effects, apply firm but mild pressure with the gua sha tool, being careful to move smoothly and fluidly over the lymphatic passages. Move outward toward the lymph nodes, starting in the middle of the face or body and going behind the ears, under the jawline, and along the collarbones. Frequent exercise promotes healthy circulation and lymphatic flow, which improves skin texture visibly and minimizes the look of puffiness and dark circles. Beginners who incorporate gua sha into their daily self-care routines report feeling more energized, with increased lymphatic drainage and improved circulation.

BENEFITS OF SKIN HEALTH

With so many advantages for skin health, gua sha therapy is a great complement to skincare regimens for novices looking for safe, efficient solutions to improve their complexion. The gua sha tool's mild scraping action encourages blood flow beneath the skin's surface, which helps skin cells receive oxygen and nutrients. A more youthful appearance is encouraged by the skin's improved suppleness and nourishment as a result of the increased circulation. Gua sha promotes collagen formation by increasing blood flow, which over time may help to lessen the appearance of fine lines and wrinkles.

Frequent gua sha treatment promotes lymphatic drainage, which helps tone facial muscles and lessens puffiness. By removing toxins and stagnant fluids from the face tissues, the little pressure used during the scraping motion helps to minimize swelling and encourage a more defined facial contour. In addition to making under-eye bags less noticeable, this lymphatic drainage action can help you have a more even, brighter complexion. Beginners might see noticeable improvements in their skin's brightness and texture by adding gua sha into their skincare routine.

Use a light facial oil or serum to make a smooth surface for the gua sha tool to glide over to optimize the health advantages of gua sha for your skin. Start by applying light strokes around the facial contours, paying particular attention to the forehead, cheeks, and jawline—areas that are prone to stress or puffiness. To promote circulation and lymphatic drainage, use upward and outward motions. Use a moisturizer to maintain the skin's natural barrier function and seal in moisture after a session. Using the restorative powers of gua sha therapy, novices can attain radiant, healthier-looking skin with regular practice.

RELAXATION AND STRESS REDUCTION

Gua sha therapy is a great option for newcomers looking for all-natural ways to decompress and enhance their general well-being because it has significant advantages for both stress relief and relaxation. The gua sha tool's mild scraping motion encourages the release of muscular tension and increases blood flow, which helps to reduce the physical signs of stress such as jaw, shoulder, and neck tightness. By triggering the body's parasympathetic nerve system, which promotes calm and lowers the release of stress chemicals, this treatment approach promotes deep relaxation.

Frequent gua sha sessions can improve brain circulation and oxygen delivery to brain cells, which can help reduce anxiety symptoms and enhance mental clarity. The gua sha tool is useful for reducing everyday stress and enhancing emotional well-being because of its rhythmic action on the skin, which produces a calming sensation that encourages mindfulness and relaxation. Beginners may find that adding gua sha to their self-care regimen offers a soothing ritual that encourages rest and aids in reestablishing mental and physical equilibrium.

To benefit from gua sha's ability to reduce stress, establish a calm, distraction-free space and gently massage your face and body's muscles with the gua sha instrument. To promote relaxation and reduce muscular tension, concentrate on the areas with the greatest amount of tension, such as the forehead, jawline, and temples.

Use slow, deliberate strokes in these areas. During gua sha treatments, incorporate deep breathing exercises to help you relax and find inner peace. Through the therapeutic benefits of gua sha, beginners can experience long-lasting stress alleviation and develop a deeper connection to their body's natural rhythms with constant practice.

IMPROVING ORGANIC DETOXIFICATION METHODS

Through lymphatic drainage and circulation enhancement, gua sha therapy helps the body's natural detoxification processes, which are essential for eliminating toxins and metabolic waste from the tissues. Gua sha tools gently scrape the body to encourage lymphatic flow, which helps transfer toxins and stagnant fluids toward lymph nodes where they can be processed and expelled from the body. This cleansing action promotes general health and vigor, lowers inflammation, and enhances cellular performance.

By stimulating the removal of excess fluids and toxins from the tissues, regular gua sha practice can help to produce a more uniform skin texture and lessen the appearance of cellulite. Increased blood flow to the skin's surface aids in the elimination of free radicals and other contaminants that can hasten the aging process and cause damage to the skin. Gua sha therapy supports the body's natural cleansing processes and, for beginners, improves energy levels, better skin, and overall well-being by strengthening the body's detoxification pathways.

Use a strong yet mild pressure with the gua sha tool, concentrating on areas like the thighs, belly, and underarms that are prone to congestion and fluid retention, to maximize the purifying effects of gua sha. As comfort permits, progressively increase pressure from soft to firm strokes, resulting in a delicate yet therapeutic experience. Drink plenty of water and include foods high in nutrients in your diet to aid in the body's detoxification process and improve your general health. Beginners can make use of the cleansing properties of gua sha therapy to support long-term health and wellness, encourage better skin, and reduce inflammation with regular practice.

CHAPTER FOUR

GETTING GUA SHA STARTED

SELECTING THE BEST GUA SHA INSTRUMENT FOR NOVICES

For beginners in particular, choosing the right Gua Sha instrument is essential to a successful session. To begin with, choose tools crafted from premium materials such as rose quartz or jade, which are renowned for their resilience and calming qualities. Additionally, these materials hold heat effectively, which improves the massage sensation. Take into account the tool's size and shape; a larger tool is more appropriate for larger body sections like the back, while a smaller tool may be easier to use in facial areas.

Another consideration is the comfort of grasp; ergonomically designed equipment guarantees easy handling during the exercise. To minimize skin discomfort or scratches, beginners might often benefit from using instruments with rounded edges.

Set aside things that you find both visually pleasing and useful, as this will motivate you to incorporate Gua Sha into your practice.

HOW TO GET READY FOR A GUA SHA SESSION

For best results, prepare your skin before beginning a Gua Sha session. To start, give your face and body a thorough cleaning to get rid of any makeup, debris, or extra oil. This guarantees that there are no obstacles in the way of the Gua Sha tool's smooth glide across your skin. To maximize skin penetration and stimulate circulation before receiving a facial Gua Sha, think about administering a mild exfoliation.

To make the Gua Sha tool's surface smooth, apply an appropriate face oil or serum. The oil improves the tool's ability to facilitate lymphatic drainage and lessen puffiness by lowering friction and enabling smooth movement. Before you start, take a moment to unwind and breathe deeply to create a peaceful environment that will support the healing effects of gua sha.

FUNDAMENTAL METHODS AND APPROACHES

To reap the full benefits of Gua Sha, beginners must first learn the fundamental practices. Start by gently tracing the natural curves of your face or body with upward strokes. Apply light to moderate pressure while making sure you are comfortable and preventing any soreness or bruises. Start in the middle of your face and work your way outward to the hairline, or in the opposite direction, from the middle of your body to the extremities.

Investigate various stroke patterns, such as lifting, rolling, and scraping motions, to efficiently target particular locations. Concentrate on regions like the jawline, neck, shoulders, or lower back that are prone to tension or stagnation. As you get more practice with the method, gently increase the pressure based on your comfort level and skin sensitivity.

Regular practice and consistency in technique will improve your proficiency and the overall health advantages of Gua Sha.

CHOOSING THE OPTIMAL LOCATION AND TIME FOR GUA SHA

The efficacy and assimilation of your Gua Sha practice into your routine are greatly influenced by the time and location you choose. Choose a peaceful, cozy area where you can unwind and concentrate without interruptions. Take into consideration adding Gua Sha to your skincare regimen, either as part of a relaxing wind-down ritual in the evening or in the morning to revitalize and depuff your face.

Make sure there is enough lighting in the area of your choice so that you can see clearly and the atmosphere is calm. Try out several times of the day to see what suits your schedule and is most effective for you. Maintaining a regular schedule is essential to establishing Gua Sha as a helpful self-care practice.

INCLUDING GUA SHA IN YOUR EVERYDAY ACTIVITIES

Including gua sha in your daily regimen can have long-term positive effects on your skin and general health. Begin by dedicating a specific period, even if it's only a few minutes, to practicing Gua Sha every day. To optimize its therapeutic effects, think about combining it with other skincare routines or self-care activities.

For convenience, keep your Gua Sha tool next to your nightstand or readily accessible in your skincare kit. Developing a routine facilitates the formation of a habit, which in turn facilitates the gradual realization of the advantages of increased lymphatic drainage, diminished puffiness, and improved circulation. To keep yourself motivated and consistent in your Gua Sha practice, keep an eye on your progress and modify your regimen as necessary.

CHAPTER FIVE

METHODS AND APPROACHES

COMPREHENSIVE HOW-TO GUIDE FOR FACE GUA SHA

A traditional Chinese treatment called facial gua sha uses gentle skin scraping to enhance lymphatic drainage, circulation, and general skin health. Applying a facial oil or serum to a clean face will help lubricate the instrument. Start in the middle of the face and carefully scrape outward and upward along the jawline while holding the Gua Sha tool flat on the skin. Apply light to medium pressure to prevent pain or bruises. For maximum effect, repeat each stroke five to ten times.

Proceed to the forehead and, to encourage face muscle relaxation and lessen tension lines, use the curved edge of the tool to scrape from the center towards the hairline. Use the smaller, curved end of the Gua Sha tool on the area under the eyes, gliding softly from the inner corner towards the temples.

This lessens dark circles and puffiness. Lastly, use a light scrape along the neck to promote lymphatic drainage. Frequent face Gua Sha use can boost the absorption of skincare products, improve skin tone, and lessen wrinkles.

METHODS FOR TARGETING VARIOUS BODY PARTS

Gua Sha is beneficial for many areas of the body and is not just for facial therapy. Use a flat stone or a broader Gua Sha instrument for the neck and shoulders. Massage oil should be applied to the skin, and the neck should be softly scraped upwards from the base to the jawline. This encourages relaxation by easing stiffness and tension.

To improve circulation and lessen muscle soreness, apply longer, sweeping strokes with the tool on the arms and legs. Make sure the pressure is firm enough to be useful but not uncomfortable by adjusting it to your comfort level. When working on particular regions, such as the thighs or calves concentrate on any sore spots and use shorter strokes to release tension.

Use a handle-equipped Gua Sha tool for greater reach when working on the back. Apply massage oil, then move from the spine outward to the shoulders and hips with long, strong strokes along the back's muscles. This method can aid with general relaxation, muscular knot reduction, and posture improvement.

PRESSURE ADJUSTMENT BASED ON COMFORT LEVELS

It's important to modify the pressure during a gua sha for maximum comfort and effectiveness. To get the skin warmed up and ready for the scraping sensation, apply gentle pressure at first. Increase the pressure gradually as you get more comfortable to boost circulation and penetrate deeper tissue layers. Avoid applying too much pressure, though, as this could result in pain or bruises.

Pay attention to the feedback that your body is giving you; if something seems sensitive or sore, slightly lessen the pressure applied. To prevent irritation, use gentle, deliberate motions when scraping rather than quick, jerky movements. Gua Sha should not hurt; rather, it should feel soothing and healing. Put varied amounts of pressure on different parts of the body. For example, put less pressure on the face and more pressure on larger muscle groups for a deeper massage.

RECOGNIZING THE STROKES' DIRECTION

To get the intended therapeutic results, Gua Sha's stroke direction is very important. Always use upward and outward strokes to promote circulation and lymphatic drainage. Move toward the bodily part's periphery starting at its core. This orientation encourages detoxification and decreases fluid retention by supporting the body's natural fluid movement.

Stroking against a muscle or joint's natural grain should be avoided since this might lead to pain or damage.

To elevate facial muscles and lessen drooping, move your hand upward along the forehead and jawline. When treating the body, follow the natural curves of the muscles and bones, modifying the tool's angle to suit the specific shape of the affected area. The therapeutic effects of Gua Sha are enhanced and a safe and effective therapy is ensured when the strokes are performed consistently and correctly.

GUA SHA IN COMBINATION WITH OTHER SKINCARE METHODS

Gua Sha's advantages can be increased by incorporating it into your skincare regimen. As a first step, cleanse and tone your skin to get it ready for treatment.

To help the instrument slide more smoothly, lubricate it with a face oil or serum. To enhance product absorption and encourage lymphatic drainage, begin with facial Gua Sha. Proceed with mild tapping or acupressure to enhance blood flow and alleviate tension in the facial muscles.

Apply your usual skincare products, such as sunscreen or moisturizer, after Gua Sha to lock in moisture and shield the skin. Gua Sha can be used in conjunction with massage or dry brushing techniques for body treatments to improve detoxification and circulation. For optimal effects, include Gua Sha in your routine two to three times a week, varying the frequency according to your skin's reaction.

You can establish a comprehensive strategy for skin health and wellness by integrating gua sha with other skincare techniques. Frequent practice enhances your skin's appearance while also fostering calm and general well-being.

CHAPTER SIX

FREQUENTLY ASKED QUESTIONS

IS EVERYONE SECURE IN GUA SHA?

When done properly, gua sha, an age-old Chinese therapeutic method, is harmless for most people. There are a few things to bear in mind, though. First and foremost, it's imperative to apply light pressure with the appropriate technique to prevent applying too much force to the skin, which may irritate or bruise it. Before attempting Gua Sha, anyone with specific medical issues, such as blood disorders or skin infections, should speak with a healthcare provider to be sure it's safe for them.

Additionally, pregnant women should concentrate on safer areas like the arms and legs rather than the lower back and abdomen when performing Gua Sha. To reduce any negative responses, it's best to test a small area beforehand and use a hypoallergenic oil or balm during the procedure for people with sensitive skin or a history of allergies.

Most people can safely enjoy the advantages of Gua Sha as long as they approach it thoughtfully and take into account any unique health considerations.

IS GUA SHA ABLE TO CREATE BRUISES?

One possible negative effect of Gua Sha is bruising, particularly if the skin is extremely sensitive or if the method is done too firmly. However, by applying light to moderate pressure and making sure the instrument slides smoothly over the skin rather than violently scraping it, bruising can be generally prevented. Utilizing a lubricant, like oil or balm, is also necessary to lower friction and facilitate the Gua Sha tool's movement.

Bruising can be avoided by beginning with shorter sessions for novices and progressively increasing the duration and pressure as they get more comfortable. Additionally, the risk of skin harm can be reduced by selecting the proper Gua Sha instrument, such as one made of rose quartz or smooth jade. People can reap the benefits of Gua Sha without having to worry about the unpleasant side effects of bruising if they practice it carefully and attentively.

HOW OFTEN SHOULD ONE PERFORM GUA SHA EXERCISES?

Gua Sha's practice frequency varies based on personal requirements and objectives. It is advised that novices begin with 1-2 sessions per week to give their skin time to adjust and avoid overstimulation. More pronounced benefits can be obtained by progressively increasing to two or three sessions per week as one grows more used to the method and its effects.

It's critical to pay attention to how your skin reacts both during and after each treatment. Any redness or soreness could indicate that you should temporarily cut back on the frequency or intensity of your Gua Sha practice. Long-term benefits require consistency, so creating a regular regimen that suits your lifestyle and skin type is crucial. In the end, each person has a different ideal frequency for practicing gua sha, and tailoring the practice to each person's feedback guarantees a secure and productive session.

WHAT OUTCOMES ARE TYPICAL OF PRACTICING GUA SHA REGULARLY?

Frequent Gua Sha practice has several possible advantages for the skin and general health. Improved circulation is one of the most obvious benefits, and it can result in a more radiant complexion and less puffiness. Over time, the gentle scraping motion of the gua sha can also aid in relaxing the muscles in the face, which can minimize the appearance of fine lines and encourage a more youthful appearance.

Gua Sha is also said to promote lymphatic drainage, which helps remove extra fluid and toxins from the face. This may lead to less puffiness beneath the eyes and a more defined jawline. After a Gua Sha session, many practitioners also report feeling calmer and less agitated because the practice encourages relaxation and calmness throughout the body.

HANDLING ALLERGIES AND SENSITIVE SKIN

It's crucial to exercise caution when performing Gua Sha on people who have sensitive skin or allergies to prevent any negative effects. Before utilizing the Gua Sha instrument, lubricating the skin with a hypoallergenic oil or balm can help decrease inflammation and reduce friction. It is also advised to test a tiny section of skin before beginning a full session to make sure the selected products work well with your skin type.

Furthermore, shielding sensitive skin from needless irritation throughout the procedure is the use of moderate pressure and gentle strokes. Avoiding broken or irritated skin is advised, and any discomfort or redness that would suggest that the method or items being used need to be changed should be noted. Benefits from Gua Sha can be safely and efficiently experienced by addressing it with sensitivity and awareness of certain skin issues.

CHAPTER SEVEN

ADVANCED METHODS FOR GUA SHA

EXAMINING CUSTOMIZED GUA SHA INSTRUMENTS

Specialized Gua Sha tools provide greater accuracy and efficacy in the procedure compared to conventional approaches. Gua Sha boards made of rose quartz or jade are common tools because of their easy-to-use smooth surfaces that promote lymphatic drainage and reduce inflammation. To provide the best pressure and comfort during treatment, these instruments are made to precisely suit the features of the face or body. Compared to makeshift tools, their ergonomic form allows practitioners to accomplish deeper tissue manipulation and greater outcomes.

Understanding the distinct uses and advantages of specialist tools is necessary before using them. For example, a Gua Sha tool with a notched edge may more successfully target acupressure sites, easing muscle tension and increasing circulation.

For bigger areas like the back or thighs, the smooth edge of a flat instrument works well for scraping, which helps to reduce cellulite and promote detoxification. By choosing instruments that fit their needs and tastes, beginners can improve their technique and guarantee a relaxing and productive Gua Sha session.

When using specific Gua Sha tools, one must practice the correct technique and modify pressure according to one's comfort level. These techniques can increase circulation, decrease puffiness, and improve skincare product absorption when added to regular skincare or wellness routines.

Practitioners can experience a revitalizing practice that promotes general well-being, whether they choose to use a jade tool for its balancing benefits or a rose quartz Gua Sha for its cooling qualities.

METHODS FOR PARTICULAR MEDICAL CONDITIONS

The focused benefits of gua sha procedures can be used for a wide range of health concerns. Using a Gua Sha instrument to scrape the affected area helps release tightness and improves blood flow to areas of discomfort and tension in the muscles. This method works well for ailments like headaches, stiff necks, and persistent back discomfort. To effectively relieve discomfort and facilitate healing, practitioners might use moderate pressure and gradually increase intensity.

By increasing collagen synthesis and boosting lymphatic drainage, facial Gua Sha treatments aim to improve skin tone and reduce indications of aging. A flat-edged tool used lightly will help reduce puffiness, smooth fine wrinkles, and bring back that young glow. Including this method in your regular skincare regimen can help to enhance the texture of your skin and encourage a clearer complexion.

Gua Sha can be administered to specific face spots to improve drainage and reduce pressure for conditions such as allergies or sinus congestion. To support the body's natural healing processes and reduce symptoms, practitioners might gently scrape along the meridian channels linked to certain diseases. Comprehending the fundamentals underlying every strategy enables novices to proficiently customize Gua Sha procedures to their health requirements.

COMBINING ACUPUNCTURE AND ACUPRESSURE WITH GUA SHA

Combining acupressure and acupuncture with gua sha improves the therapeutic effects of traditional Chinese medicine. Practitioners can address a wide range of health issues, including stress alleviation, emotional balance, and chronic pain management, by integrating different modalities. While Gua Sha treatments assist in alleviating muscle tension and increase circulation along meridional pathways, acupuncture needles target specific acupuncture points.

Similar to the scraping motion used in Gua Sha, acupressure applies pressure to particular places on the body without the use of equipment. Acupressure practitioners can enhance the benefits of both techniques—deeper relaxation and pain relief—by adding Gua Sha into their sessions. A more individualized treatment plan that takes into account each patient's preferences and health goals is made possible by this integrated approach.

Acupuncturists and Gua Sha practitioners together can provide holistic treatment for both physical and energy problems. These methods can be deliberately combined to enhance holistic wellness and maximize treatment outcomes.

To achieve successful healing and well-being, those who are new to this integration may find it helpful to consult with licensed practitioners who are aware of the synergies between acupuncture, acupressure, and Gua Sha.

ADVANCED METHODS FOR GETTING A GUA SHA

Complex techniques that target specific parts of the face to increase relaxation and regeneration are used in advanced facial Gua Sha practices. Usually, these procedures start with a mild cleanse and tone to get the skin ready for the therapy. Practitioners apply gentle, controlled strokes around the jawline, cheeks, and forehead with a flat-edged Gua Sha tool to encourage lymphatic drainage and minimize puffiness.

Light, repeated strokes are used in techniques like feathering to promote collagen formation and enhance skin flexibility.

Expert practitioners can use sculpting motions to minimize the look of tiny wrinkles and define facial contours. They can tailor treatments to target specific issues like drooping skin or uneven texture by modifying the pressure and changing the angle of the stroke.

Techniques that target particular organ system-related meridian points as part of a facial Gua Sha program can also help to promote general health and vigor. Including these techniques in your regular skincare routine improves the way products absorb into your skin and promotes long-term skin health. Novices can become proficient in advanced face Gua Sha by practicing under the supervision of more seasoned practitioners or by following tutorials that prioritize safety and correct technique.

ADDING SERUMS AND ESSENTIAL OILS FOR INCREASED BENEFITS

By feeding the skin and promoting relaxation, adding essential oils and serums to Gua Sha treatments increases the therapeutic advantages. To enhance the effects of aromatherapy and elevate mood, essential oils such as lavender or rosemary can be applied topically to the skin and diluted with a carrier oil before a Gua Sha treatment. These oils are also anti-inflammatory, which enhances the cleansing benefits of gua sha.

During a Gua Sha treatment, serums rich in vitamins and antioxidants can be gently massaged into the skin to promote moisture and fight the effects of aging. A Gua Sha tool's smooth gliding motion aids in the uniform distribution of various compositions, enhancing absorption and effectiveness. Professionals can select serums that are specific to their skin type and problems; for example, they can select brightening formulas or wrinkle-minimizing ones.

Incorporating Gua Sha practices with essential oils and serums results in an opulent skincare routine that promotes mental and physical health. These products and procedures work in concert to create a bright complexion and a calming sense of well-being. To create a customized and efficient skincare routine, novices can try out various oil and serum combinations to see what suits their skin type the best.

CHAPTER EIGHT

GUA SHA FOR REJUVENATION OF THE FACE

BENEFITS OF FACIAL GUA SHA FOR ANTI-AGING

Facial Gua Sha is well known for its anti-aging properties, providing a safe, all-natural method of skin rejuvenation. Using a smooth-edged tool to gently scrape the skin's surface increases blood circulation, which in turn promotes the supply of nutrients and oxygen to the skin cells? Over time, this improved circulation aids in lessening the visibility of wrinkles and fine lines.

Additionally, the method promotes lymphatic drainage, which helps eliminate toxins and lessen puffiness, both of which can give the illusion of younger skin.

Frequent use of facial gua sha can increase the production of collagen, which is essential for preserving the firmness and flexibility of the skin.

This increase in collagen helps to improve the overall texture and smoothness of the skin. Gua Sha sessions can relieve stress and prevent the production of expression lines by gently pressing on the facial muscles. Gua Sha is a holistic technique that encourages relaxation, which can lessen the appearance of wrinkles and frown lines caused by stress.

The key to maximizing the anti-aging effects of facial gua sha is to use a light hand and stick to a regular schedule. To make the surface of your skin smooth enough for the tool to glide over, start with a clean face and add some serum or oil. Concentrating on regions prone to drooping and wrinkles, start from the neck and work your way up to the forehead with light, upward strokes. Over time, adding two to three times a week of Facial Gua Sha to your skincare routine can produce dramatic benefits in the elasticity, texture, and tone of your skin.

METHODS FOR DIMINISHING FINE LINES AND WRINKLES

Specific techniques are used in facial gua sha to naturally decrease wrinkles and fine lines. Wrinkles can be minimized and smoothed out with a Gua Sha instrument, like jade or rose quartz scraper, by gently working on the skin. The secret is to go always upwards and outwards with firm yet delicate strokes to improve circulation and lymphatic drainage. Through improved skin hydration and suppleness, this approach not only helps to minimize existing wrinkles but also keeps new ones from emerging.

Concentrating on regions where wrinkles are more likely to appear, like the nasolabial folds, forehead lines, and the area around the eyes (crow's feet), is one useful method. To encourage the formation of collagen and enhance the firmness of your skin, lightly scrape along these lines with the curved edge of the Gua Sha tool while applying minimal pressure. Feathering is another useful method that improves oxygenation and blood flow across the face with quick, gentle strokes. Over time, this helps to fill up the skin and lessen the depth of fine wrinkles.

For best outcomes, you need to be consistent. Include a facial gua sha in your skincare regimen two or three times a week at the very least. To improve the tool's smoother movements and better skin absorption, pair it with moisturizing serums or oils.

To guarantee that your Gua Sha tool continues to help keep youthful-looking skin, remember to clean it after every use to avoid bacterial development.

IMPROVING ELASTICITY AND CONTOURS OF THE FACE

The benefits of face gua sha include improving skin suppleness and facial features naturally. Your face can be molded to look more like it has more definition by using a Gua Sha tool to gently manipulate the skin. The method entails lifting and firming the skin, especially around the jawline, cheeks, and temples, with the tool's curved edges.

This promotes a more youthful facial structure and tones the muscles underneath.

Start by lubricating the skin with a face oil or serum to guarantee smooth tool glide and effectively enhance facial contours. Using light, upward strokes, start in the middle of the face, close to the chin or nose, and work your way outward to the hairline or ears. Concentrate on the regions where you want to draw attention to the definition of the contours like the cheekbones for a more sculpted look or the jawline to lift sagging skin.

Through the stimulation of collagen formation and the enhancement of blood flow to the skin cells, facial gua sha also helps to improve skin flexibility. Improved oxygenation and nutrition delivery are made possible by this increase in circulation, which is crucial for keeping skin firm and supple. Frequent use of facial gua sha can improve overall youthfulness and vitality by preventing sagging and encouraging a more toned facial structure over time.

GUA SHA TIPS FOR GLOWING SKIN

It takes more than just the facial gash method to get bright skin; you also need to incorporate the proper practices into your skincare regimen. To begin, select a premium Gua Sha instrument crafted from rose quartz, jade, or similar silky material that is easy to apply to the skin. Make sure your face is clean before starting a Gua Sha session, and use a serum or oil to add hydration and slide.

Use slow, moderate strokes to encourage lymphatic drainage and blood circulation during the Gua Sha session. Pay attention to regions that are prone to dullness, like the forehead, cheekbones, and under the eyes. Toxins are eliminated, and a healthy glow is encouraged from within. Use feathering techniques to reenergize your skin by increasing blood flow and oxygenation with quick, light strokes across your face.

The secret to getting and keeping radiant skin with facial gua sha is consistency. Try to use this method two or three times a week, varying the pressure and pace of your strokes according to the toleration and sensitivity of your skin. Apply a moisturizer or extra serum after every Gua Sha treatment to seal in hydration and get the most out of it. You'll see enhanced skin luminosity, smoother texture, and a natural, healthy glow with consistent practice.

FIGHTING DARK CIRCLES AND PUFFINESS

Facial Gua Sha provides practical methods for addressing dark circles and puffiness, which are issues that many people have. Gua Sha improves blood circulation and lymphatic drainage, which helps lessen fluid retention and puffiness around the eyes and face. The lymphatic system is stimulated by the light scraping motion, which helps to eliminate toxins and extra fluid that cause puffiness.

The curved edges of the Gua Sha tool should be used with delicate yet forceful strokes to properly alleviate puffiness. With mild pressure, work your way outward toward the temples from the inner corners of the eyes to promote drainage.

To aid in reducing swelling and promoting a more lifted appearance, repeat this motion multiple times.

Facial gua sha can also help with dark circles because it can increase oxygenation and circulation. To assist release trapped blood and lessen the look of dark circles, gently massage the region beneath your eyes using the rounded edge of the Gua Sha instrument. For optimal effects, include this in your nightly skincare routine. Make sure to stick with it to sustain over time brighter, more refreshed under-eye skin.

You may use the natural benefits of facial gua sha to reduce dark circles, fight puffiness, and look younger by including these strategies in your skincare routine. Facial Gua Sha's ability to support general skin health and vitality will be further enhanced by regular practice, appropriate hydration, and enough sleep.

CHAPTER NINE

GUA SHA TO ALLEVIATE PAIN

RELIEVING MIGRAINES AND TENSION HEADACHES

By encouraging improved circulation and relieving muscle tension in the head, neck, and shoulder regions, gua sha, a traditional Chinese therapy, provides relief from tension headaches and migraines. Practitioners gently scrape the skin with a smooth-edged tool to increase blood flow and lessen stiffness.

Gradually build up from a light pressure point by following the curves of your forehead, temples, and base of the skull. This method works well for both preventing and treating headaches because it releases tension that has built up and promotes general relaxation.

To relieve the pain and promote blood circulation in the temporal zones of your migraine, gently scrape in an outward motion. To stop skin irritation, it's critical to apply constant pressure and refrain from overscraping. To effectively manage headache frequency and intensity, incorporate this technique into your routine at the outset of symptoms or as a preventive strategy.

METHODS FOR TREATING SHOULDER AND NECK PAIN

Gua Sha works wonders to relieve shoulder and neck discomfort by encouraging lymphatic drainage and focusing on tense muscles. Start by applying a light coating of massage oil or balm to improve glide and lessen resistance. With the tool, move in long, sweeping motions in the direction of the heart, applying equal pressure to the shoulder and neck muscles. This method improves the range of motion and offers instant comfort by assisting in the release of knots and tightness.

Pay particular attention to the areas along your spine and in your trapezius muscles that are the most tense.

To provide a controlled and smooth scraping motion, adjust the pressure to your comfort level. Frequent practice is a great complement to alternative therapies and self-care regimens because it can greatly lessen chronic neck and shoulder pain.

REDUCING STIFFNESS AND MUSCLE SORENESS

Gua Sha works by increasing blood flow and dissolving scar tissue to relieve stiffness and discomfort in the muscles. To enable easy scraping motions, liberally apply oil or balm to the impacted region. Focusing on the tense and uncomfortable areas, move the tool in parallel strokes while applying light pressure to the tight muscles. This method facilitates the release of lactic acid accumulation and enhances muscular recuperation following strenuous exercise or extended durations of physical activity.

Focus on particular muscle areas, such as the lower back, thighs, and calves, and change the pressure until it feels comfortable for you.

Gua Sha can help you recover from a workout more quickly and maintain the general health of your muscles by improving flexibility, lowering inflammation, and preventing muscular stiffness.

GUA SHA FOR ARTHRITIS AND JOINT PAIN

Gua Sha reduces inflammation and enhances joint mobility to provide relief from arthritis and joint discomfort.

To reduce friction during scraping, start by lightly coating the afflicted joints with oil or balm. Move the tool in tiny, circular strokes along the joints while applying strong yet mild pressure. Concentrate on swollen or painful areas, like the elbows, wrists, and knees, to increase blood flow and reduce stiffness.

Keep your pressure on your pain threshold and avoid applying pressure directly to irritated joints. Frequent treatments can improve joint function and general mobility by easing the chronic pain and stiffness associated with arthritis.

Use this method regularly or as needed to help maintain joint health and lessen the severity of arthritic symptoms.

HOW TO INCLUDE GUA SHA IN PHYSICAL THERAPY PRACTICES

By focusing on lowering pain, increasing circulation, and treating muscle tightness, incorporating Gua Sha into physical therapy regimens improves treatment outcomes. Assess the patient's condition thoroughly before applying the appropriate amount of oil or balm to the treatment region.

To enhance flexibility and relieve adhesions, gently move the tool over muscles and connective tissues while applying moderate pressure.

Make an effort to include Gua Sha methods that enhance current therapies and therapeutic objectives. This could include working on certain muscle groups or improving the range of motion in joints that have been damaged or are suffering from long-term illnesses.

Frequent sessions are a useful supplement to all-encompassing physical therapy programs because they can enhance rehabilitation efforts, hasten recovery, and optimize physical function.

CHAPTER TEN

INCLUDING GUA SHA IN HEALTH-RELATED ACTIVITIES

GUA SHA USE IN STRESS REDUCTION

Traditional Chinese medicine gave rise to the age-old medicinal practice known as gua sha, which provides an effective way to control stress. With a smooth-edged tool, Gua Sha gently scrapes the skin to encourage circulation and remove built-up tension in the muscles and fascia. This procedure promotes relaxation and helps to reduce the body's reactions to stress, such as tenseness and discomfort. Gua Sha's rhythmic strokes enhance blood flow and activate the lymphatic system, which helps with detoxification and enhances general well-being.

It can be incredibly transformational to incorporate Gua Sha into your stress-reduction regimen. You'll feel a progressive release of tension and a calming sensation spreading throughout your body as you glide the tool over specific parts of your body, especially the neck, shoulders, and upper back where stress tends to gather. As you concentrate on the movements and sensations associated with this exercise, you will be able to cultivate awareness and find a natural way to decompress from every day tensions. Gua Sha is a useful supplement to any wellness routine since it promotes mental clarity and physical relaxation when used regularly for stress management.

ADVANTAGES OF GUA SHA RITUALS AT NIGHT

Rituals using Gua Sha at night have special advantages that improve the quality of your sleep and your general sense of relaxation. After a demanding day, incorporating this technique into your evening routine might aid in your physical and mental relaxation. Gua Sha's mild scraping motion encourages blood flow and eases tense muscles, setting your body up for rejuvenating slumber. Your entire body can become more relaxed and tension-free by concentrating on certain areas such as the neck, shoulders, and face.

Moreover, lymphatic drainage is encouraged by evening Gua Sha routines, which help to lessen puffiness and encourage a brighter complexion. Beyond the physical sphere, this technique has relaxing effects since deliberate movements and repetitive strokes can reduce mental stress and encourage serenity before bed. Spend some time breathing deeply and letting your thoughts relax from the day's events while you move the Gua Sha tool over your skin. In addition to improving relaxation, this thoughtful approach to self-care also prepares the body for a more restful and revitalizing sleep cycle.

USING GUA SHA IN A HOLISTIC SELF-CARE APPROACH

Gua Sha is a fundamental component of holistic self-care regimens, providing numerous advantages for the body and mind. Gua Sha fosters total well-being by integrating mind-body connection, in addition to its physical effects of improving lymphatic drainage, lowering muscle tension, and boosting circulation. Including this age-old method in your self-care regimen promotes deliberate relaxation and mindfulness. Whether you apply Gua Sha to your body, face, or certain acupressure spots, you are promoting overall balance and developing a closer relationship with your body's requirements.

Gua Sha is ideal for holistic self-care, which highlights the connection between one's physical, emotional, and spiritual well-being. By making time for this practice, you can promote long-term wellness in addition to addressing urgent issues like facial strain or muscle stiffness. Gua Sha's ritualistic elements promote introspection and mindfulness, enabling you to block out time during the day for rest and renewal. Gua Sha supports a balanced and happy existence and has holistic advantages that go well beyond the physical, whether you practice it every day or include it in weekly rituals.

GUA SHA IN CONJUNCTION WITH MINDFULNESS AND MEDITATION

The benefits of each practice are increased when Gua Sha is combined with mindfulness and meditation, producing a synergistic effect that improves general well-being. Gua Sha facilitates physical relaxation and energy flow, while meditation develops mental clarity and emotional resilience. When combined, these techniques offer a mind-body-centered approach to self-care. Set a goal for your session at the outset, be it self-nurturing, developing gratitude, or relieving tension.

Pay attention to the movements and sensations of the Gua Sha against your skin as you incorporate it into your meditation practice. Along acupressure points or tense spots, apply light, purposeful strokes, coordinating your breathing with each motion. By using a conscious approach, you can expand your meditation experience and increase the effectiveness of Gua Sha. Combining these techniques results in a soothing ritual that enhances both exterior and internal relaxation and helps you maintain harmony and balance in your day-to-day activities.

BENEFITS OF REGULAR GUA SHA PRACTICE IN THE LONG RUN

Regular Gua Sha practice has several long-term advantages that improve general health and well-being. Over time, better skin and less inflammation can be achieved by using Gua Sha to boost the body's natural cleansing processes through enhanced circulation and lymphatic drainage. The mild scraping action improves muscle tone and promotes tissue regeneration by dissolving adhesions and scar tissue. Gua Sha is a great addition to active lifestyles due to its physical benefits, which include increased flexibility, less stiffness, and improved mobility.

Moreover, consistent Gua Sha practice has significant psychological benefits. This technique's ritualistic quality encourages self-awareness and mindfulness by prompting you to check in with your body and quickly treat any areas of tension or discomfort.

Resilience and self-care get stronger as you become more aware of your body's requirements. Regular Gua Sha practice over time can help with stress reduction, better sleep, and an increased sense of general well-being. By committing to this age-old healing method, you develop a balanced and full life by investing in your current and future well-being.

CHAPTER ELEVEN
UPCOMING DEVELOPMENTS AND TRENDS

NEW DEVELOPMENTS IN GUA SHA INSTRUMENTS AND METHODS

Innovation in traditional methods has surged because of recent developments in Gua Sha tools and procedures. To better serve practitioners as well as individuals experimenting with self-care at home, contemporary Gua Sha tools now have ergonomic designs that improve usability and effectiveness. Due to their alleged energy qualities, materials like rose quartz and jade are becoming more and more well-liked, giving the practice a more comprehensive aspect. Additionally, certain equipment has pressure settings that may be adjusted to provide customized treatments, guaranteeing patient comfort and safety throughout sessions.

In terms of technique, the emphasis is increasingly on delicate application and precision to produce desired therapeutic results without creating discomfort. Gua Sha is being incorporated into skincare routines for the face and body in novel ways by practitioners, who hope to enhance collagen formation, lymphatic drainage, and general skin regeneration. These developments highlight how Gua Sha has developed from a conventional therapeutic approach to a flexible health regimen that is widely accepted.

TECHNOLOGY INTEGRATION IN GUA SHA PRACTICES

Technology is starting to play a major part in improving Gua Sha practices by fusing cutting-edge discoveries with age-old methods. These days, users can learn optimal techniques and pressure points from apps and digital guides that provide individualized routines and training. Real-time feedback on pressure and angle is provided by smart Gua Sha instruments with sensors, guaranteeing uniform and efficient treatments. This kind of integration improves each session's accuracy and therapeutic advantages in addition to making learning easier.

Additionally, advances in material science have resulted in the creation of hypoallergenic and antibacterial Gua Sha instruments that solve hygiene issues and suit sensitive skin types. Beyond personal usage, technology helps professionals in clinical settings by improving patient care outcomes, optimizing workflow, and digitizing medical data and treatment plans. These technological advancements show how Gua Sha is evolving into a contemporary, approachable wellness technique.

WORKSHOPS AND EDUCATIONAL INITIATIVES ON GUA SHA

Gua Sha seminars and educational programs have spread throughout the world, serving a wide range of students and professionals who want to improve their knowledge and abilities. Workshops give practical instruction in both traditional techniques and their modern applications, while also covering the history and tenets of Gua Sha. Participants get a deep respect for this age-old healing art by learning about various tools, their applications, and cultural variances in technique.

In addition, accessible learning alternatives such as webinars and online courses let enthusiasts study at their own pace and interact with a worldwide community of practitioners. These learning environments not only encourage the growth of skills but also stress the value of moral behavior and customer safety. Educational endeavors are vital to the preservation and innovation of Gua Sha practices for future generations, as they facilitate the sharing of knowledge and skills.

INTERNATIONAL VIEWS OF GUA SHA'S EFFECT

Gua Sha's influence is cross-cultural; its holistic approach to well-being and therapeutic advantages has led to its acceptance and recognition on a global scale.

Gua Sha is still incorporated into traditional medical practices in Asia, the region of its origin. It is used there to treat a variety of health issues, including pain management and detoxification. Gua Sha has become more well-known in Western nations' wellness spas and holistic health facilities due to its reputation for easing tension in the muscles, enhancing circulation, and encouraging relaxation.

Furthermore, a growing body of research and clinical trials is confirming the effectiveness of Gua Sha in treating a range of ailments, which is helping conventional healthcare systems adopt it.

The international exchange of knowledge via conferences, books, and online resources promotes appreciation of Gua Sha's therapeutic potential as well as cross-cultural understanding. This worldwide viewpoint highlights the function of gua sha as a cultural bridge that promotes wellness worldwide, in addition to its use as a medicinal method.

ECOLOGICAL METHODS IN GUA SHA PRODUCTION

Gua Sha manufacture has made sustainability a priority, working to reduce its negative effects on the environment and encourage the ethical source of its components. To lessen their carbon impact and encourage ethical mining methods, manufacturers are choosing more and more environmentally friendly materials, such as recycled metals and gemstones that are sourced ethically. Furthermore, the goal of improved production procedures is to reduce energy and waste during the manufacturing process.

Sustainable practices are also influenced by packaging advances, as businesses choose to use biodegradable materials and simple designs that put use over extravagance. Gua Sha manufacturing is guaranteed to have a beneficial impact on local economies and social welfare through initiatives that support fair labor practices and community engagement in the sourcing countries.